The Final Edge

Look & Feel Your Best
Winning the Weigth Loss Game

Terry Linde, C.S.C.S.

IA Publications

THE FINAL EDGE
Look & Feel Your Best-Winning the Weight Loss Game

Published by IA Publications, a division of Destiny Management.
Edited and Produced by Terry Linde.

<u>Forward</u>

In 1983, with Arnold Schwarzenegger as my inspiration, I began my career in bodybuilding. Since junior high, I knew that I wanted to dedicate my life to fitness. Attempting to emulate Arnold's determination, perseverance and dedication, I focused my college training toward bodybuilding.

With all the information I was learning, it was clear that if I listened to everybody and everything that was out there, I would be left bouncing off white padded walls. Through my education of basic principles and experimentation, I sifted through the misleading information and created a system I've successfully used in our Personal Training business for over eight years now.

With this book and video system, I hope to teach you these same principles that will enable you to achieve your fitness goals, without having to waste your valuable time on nonsense.

A sincere thank-you to my family and friends for supporting and tolerating me during this process.

CONTENTS

ABOUT THE AUTHOR

Terry Linde, President of Destiny Management, LLC., has been a Personal Trainer for the past fourteen years. He has a Bachelor of Science degree in Physical Education with a minor in Business. He also carries certifications in the NASM (National Academy of Sports Medicine), World Instructor Training Schools (WITS), and the NSCA (National Strength Coaches Association). He has worked in clubs and been involved in this industry for over 25 years. He has been involved with amateur bodybuilding and powerlifting, both as a competitor and judge, for over a decade. Terry has worked with people of all ages, backgrounds and goals.

After extensive research and the encouragement of clients and friends, he wrote The Final Edge series.   This guide is not intended to take the place of a personal trainer, because of motivational factors among others, but it will give you all the information you need to set-up an individualized routine that will absolutely ensure success.

PRECAUTIONS

It is recommended that anyone who is interested in pursuing a program of physical fitness consult their physician for a complete physical examination. This physical should include, but is not limited to: blood pressure check, heart rate check, body composition analysis, anthropometric measurements, cholesterol test, and maximal or sub-maximal stress tests, particularly for men over 40 and women over 50.

Always start slow with any program. The first few weeks are not to make great strength or conditioning gains but to establish motor patterning (coordination) for the exercises.

For resistance exercise, I recommend starting with a weight that you can comfortably get to the upper range of the recommended repetitions. Perform just one set of resistance exercises the first week. If no soreness is experienced the next two days, go to two sets the second week. Progress to three sets the third week, if again, you experience no soreness. You can then raise the weight 5 pounds every time all of the sets can be performed at the upper range with good technique. If soreness is experienced, don't add sets until you can perform without soreness two days later.

For cardiovascular exercise, start with 15 minutes in the target heart range three times per week. Add 5 minutes per week up to 60 minutes, then add one day per week up to six days per week maximum, depending on your goals.

CHAPTER 1:
GETTING STARTED

The fitness movement has caught on and is here to stay. Just like any other industry, there has developed a large base of misinformation that has been integrated with sound, scientifically based health and fitness principles. This book was written and designed to:

- provide quality information
- encourage individuals to use the system by ease of design
- provide the vital tools necessary to assist in achievement of the trainees' goals.
- separate the mass of misinformation from the facts.

Our goal is to give you access to a personal trainer at a fraction of the cost of hiring one. Using the components of our system, you will be able to design and implement a personalized system to help you achieve your goals. Keep in mind that there are four main components that lead you to fitness:

- Sound nutrition
- Progressive Resistance
- Cardiovascular exercise
- Flexibility

We've outlined the basics of these components to enable you to create a program specifically for you. The information presented to you may seem complicated, so focus on these two factors:

1) Three factors control the 'nutrition' component. These are *Total Calories:* how many calories do you eat in a day?, *Spacing:* how often are you eating? (hopefully lots!), and *Ratios:* what is the mixture of proteins, carbohydrates and fats in any given meal you eat?

2) The three variables affecting your progressive resistance and cardiovascular workouts are frequency, intensity and duration. *Frequency:* how often are you performing this activity? *Intensity:* what amount of effort are you putting into this activity? *Duration:* how long are you performing this activity? No matter what activities you choose, these are the only variables that are adjusted to reach your goals.

Personal training is a growing industry and an excellent means of maximizing one's efforts, but it is also a financial commitment. This book will provide its user accurate, scientifically based, easy to use information at a fraction of the cost of a personal trainer. Although we have tried to make this guide as easy to use and follow as possible, no two bodies respond the same way to a training program. The information contained here is presented as scientifically based guidelines, which can be easily individualized for each user's own needs.

CHAPTER 2:
SELECTING A HEALTH CLUB

Before you can get started with a physical fitness program, decide what type of equipment you want to use (freeweights, machines, Nautilus, Cybex, etc.) and where you want to train (home, health club, hard-core gym, office, etc.). The best choice for you is **the facility and equipment that fits you and your lifestyle best**, and will keep you motivated enough to continue using it on a regular basis. Making the wrong choices will keep you from continuing to workout

You should also select the *type* of equipment that you as an individual enjoy working with. While each type of equipment may look and feel different from the next, they all work the same muscle groups, so choose whatever feels best to you. Attitude and commitment are more important than equipment in achieving your goals. Many elite athletes have faced limitations and overcome them. With a positive attitude and enough determination, you can overcome any obstacle.

When selecting the type of equipment to use, the most important characteristic to look for is the proper feel of the equipment. Try it before you choose! Don't choose it just because it's supposed to be good, and a famous person endorses it. If it feels smooth and comfortable without feeling awkward it is right for *you*.

SELECTING THE TYPE OF EQUIPMENT

When making your decision, ask yourself:

1) Does it feel consistent and smooth throughout the entire range of motion? If not, move on.

2) Does it fit you comfortably? Make sure that the seat adjustments fit you, especially if you are tall, short, narrow or wide.

3) Does it apply too much resistance at the beginning and not at the end or vice versa? If yes, try another.

4) Are there any sticking points? Any points throughout the range of motion where it is not smooth or tension is not being applied equally. If yes, it's not for you.
5) Is it well maintained? Particularly when selecting a health club, it is very important (whether it be for your safety or the achievement of your goals) that the equipment is maintained properly.
6) Does it hurt your joints or limit you in any way? If yes, don't consider this one.

SELECTING THE TYPE OF CLUB

In selecting a health club you should consider the following:

1)   *What type of club do you prefer?*

        a) Hard-core - Mostly bodybuilders and power lifters. High on atmosphere, low on luxury and member pampering.

        b) Fitness - All types of people serious about getting healthy. Service oriented and semi-luxurious.

        c) Social - For those who prefer to mingle. Very large, comfortable places with juice bars, lounges, etc.

2)   *What amenities are you looking for?* There should be lockers and hairdryers provided in the locker rooms, and possibly towel service as well. Tanning and massage are very popular. Ask about child care.

3)   *What fits into your budget the best?* The more amenities, the higher the cost. They should also be willing to let you try the club at no cost or apply a walk-in fee towards your membership. Try to visit t he club for a few days before deciding if it is for you.

4)   *Distance from home or office?* It should be convenient to get to at all times and on all days.

5)   *How long has the club been in business?* If you buy a long-term membership, the club might not be around for the length of your membership. If you are going to make a large investment as found I n an extended year plan, find out as much as you can about its financial solvency. Ask for some hard figures, and what ifs (what if the club closes prior to the end of your membership?)

6)   *What is their total membership?* How many of the members are active? Inactive? There may be a reason. Some clubs, especially the larger ones, might be reluctant to give out this information. Explain to them that this information is mportant in helping you to make up your mind about the club. With highly advertised clubs membership size might be a problem when trying to use the equipment when you want to. This information is vital.

7)   *Does this club use high-pressure sales tactics?*   If so, you might spend more time upgrading your membership options   than actually working out.

8)   *Is there enough equipment to handle the current membership, and I s the equipment well maintained?*   If there are lines to use the equipment, you may find it very difficult to get a good workout.

When taking your tour of the facility, look at the condition of the equipment. Are there many pieces out of   service? Are the pads needing replacement?   Do the machines look like they need r eplacing?

9)   *How busy are they during peak hours?* Usually peak hours include 5:30 a.m. -7:00 a.m., 11:30 a.m.-1:00 p.m., and 4:00 p.m.-7:00 p.m. make sure you make it a point to visit the club during the time you most likely will be using it. This will give you a good feel for how busy it is and what kinds of lines, if any, you might encounter.

10)   *What about employee participation?* Are their employees knowledgeable and helpful? Are they certified? If not, be wary of advice. Are the employees active participants? They should help as spotters, coaches, and encourage you to perform at your best every workout. Are there enough employees   to   handle   the membership? It does no good if no one has the time for you.

ALTERNATIVES TO HEALTH CLUBS

If you don't want to fight all the people, don't have the extra time to drive to a gym, or just can't find a facility to suit your needs, a home gym is the best idea. However, keep in mind that unless you have the money to invest in a well-equipped home gym, a commercial gym will offer more variety and safety.

CHAPTER 3:
DIET AND NUTRITION

Nutrition is over 50% of the fitness battle. A vital aspect of better health, is the need to maintain a level of basic nutrition. In an attempt to achieve their goals, people will often try everything in sight. Calories will be drastically reduced in an effort to lose weight while the person seeking weight gain will gorge themselves. Neither is healthy nor permanent. Following are ways to achieve both fat loss and lean gain goals using the three components of nutrition.

CALORIES

<u>FAT LOSS</u>

Particularly appealing are the fad diets that promise to help you lose weight in a very short period of time. These diets try to help you by drastically reducing your caloric intake to lose "weight" fast.

Although this process may be successful at first, it does have very serious drawbacks. The reason fad diets are not the way to go in order to lose fat and keep it off are three fold:

1)	Metabolism (the number of calories your body burns per day) is slowed, as muscle is lost along with fat and water.

2)	Fad diets only work for a limited time. As your body loses muscle, your metabolism slows down until you can only burn the number of calories you're consuming on the diet.

3)	Low-calorie diets do not provide enough nutrients for you to stay healthy.

The average person can use 2200-2500 calories per day to maintain weight without any additional activity. The main need for these calories comes from lean body mass (muscle). If you cut the calories by more than 500 per day, the metabolism will slow down. As an example: If you are able to burn 2,500 calories per day and you are only taking in 1,000 calories per day, your metabolism will slow down until you can only burn 1,000 calories per day instead of 2,500 calories. Your metabolism does this by utilizing your lean body mass for energy, as only the muscles require calories at rest. Then, as you are losing muscle, and burning fewer calories per day, you have to keep cutting the calories more to lose more. Then, just when you thought things were perfect, you got rid of the "weight", and you start eating your regular caloric intake, you gain the weight right back. Why? Because now that your metabolism is lowered, any time you eat more than the previous calorie level (which is easy to do because the fad diets are usually not higher than 1,000 calories per day), the extra calories will be stored as fat.

Another problem is the fact that your system has been gearing up to store body fat by increasing the efficiency of certain enzymes that promote body fat storage. The body reacts this way because it believes it is starving and needs to store fat as a reserve source of energy.

Historically, this storage system is what has helped protect us in times of famine and helped us continue the human race. Fortunately, famines are not a problem that most of us deal with today, but if we diet this way our bodies still retain body fat thus resulting in the 'Yo-Yo' syndrome of dieting. Almost all people who lose weight gain it back within 5 years; they usually gain back all of the weight they lost - plus some! Every time this process occurs, the metabolism is damaged. So what do you do?

As you have probably figured out, when trying to achieve basic, healthy nutrition, you must stay away from anything that promises changes in a short period of time. If it has taken years for you to get the way you are, it will take at least a couple of years to undo what has already been done. Physiologically, the maximum you can lose is two pounds of fat per week, (on average) as the body is unable to properly process more than this. Any more weight loss than two pounds per week would be water and muscle.

The ideal way to lose fat and keep it off is to reduce your calories slightly, and increase your activity. The maximum you should reduce your intake is by 500 calories per day and increasing activity by 500 calories per day. This will provide you a 1,000 calorie deficit per day and a loss of two pounds per week. (One pound of fat is equal to 3,500 calories; 1000 calories multiplied by seven days is 7000 calories, thus a loss of two pounds of fat per week.). Since we cannot determine how your metabolism has been affected by previous dieting, and since this is not a perfect world, a more realistic fat-loss anticipation is one pound per week.

LEAN GAIN

If you thought fat-loss was slow, be prepared to acquire even more patience for muscle gain. Gorging yourself with calories is not the correct way to gain weight unless you want to gain fat. Resistance training is critical to gaining the correct weight - MUSCLE WEIGHT!

For a beginner, a two to four pound gain in muscle per month is not uncommon. Once you have been lifting for a while (more than six months) one pound of lean body mass gain per month is excellent, and one pound of lean mass every other month is more realistic. This is roughly six pounds per year.

Since one pound of muscle is equal to 600 calories, you don't need to raise calories as drastically as you reduce them for fat. From maintenance levels, simply add 100-200 calories per day. Some hard gainers may need to add more, but this should be a good start.

Body composition testing (see chapter 9) should be done monthly to ensure your weight gain is lean. If you are not gaining lean after the first month of adding 100-200 calories above maintenance, add an additional 50 calories per day until you find that correct level for weight gain. Whether weight loss or weight gain is desired, determine how many calories per day you require for the quickest results.

HOW MANY CALORIES PER DAY SHOULD I EAT?

The equation to use is as follows:

[Body weight (in kg) x 24] - [body weight (in kg) x 0.1 x # of hours of sleep per night] + [body weight (in lbs.) x activity factor* x hours of activity] + 10% of total

Explanation:

1)   Divide your current body weight by 2.2 (to convert it to kilograms). This =___________(A)

2)   Multiply (A) by 24 (for hours in the day).
        This =___________(B)

3)   Multiply (A) by 0.1, then multiply that number by the number of hours of sleep you get per night. This   =___________ (C).

4)   Subtract (C) from (B). This =_______________(D).

5)   Multiply your body weight in pounds by the activity factor (see chart of examples of activity factors), then multiply times the hours of activity in your day. This =___________(E).

*For a more exact count, you need to break down your daily activity by the hour and use a different activity factor for each hour. However, it is easier just to average the days activities (pick a number that averages all of the activities you do in a day) and make individual adjustments afterwards.

6)   Add (D) to (E). This =___________(F).

7)   Multiply (F) by 1.1 to add for the influence of food   (calories required during digestion). This   =_______________(G).

8)   (G) is the number of calories you require to maintain your current body weight. To reduce your current weight to your desired   goal you will need to follow the 500/500 formula of reducing the number of calories you consume by 500 and increasing the number of calories of activity by 500.

Examples of activity factors:

rest (lying still, reading)	0.23
very light (sewing, singing, standing, studying)	0.27
light (office work, dish washing, shopping)	0.36
moderate (golf, nursing, housekeeping)	0.50
severe (dancing, walking 3-4 mph)	0.77
very severe (running, walking 5 mph)	1.03

The above formula provides you a rough idea of your calorie requirement per day. There will need to be some adjustments, as normally you would not maintain the same activity factor throughout the day and individual differences are not taken into consideration. Also, the formula uses your total body weight. As discussed earlier, muscle is the only thing that requires calories at rest. So, to be more accurate you should have your lean body mass determined with a body composition test (discussed in chapter 9).

A final consideration is your current diet and at what level your metabolism is currently at (if it is functioning optimally or if it is slowed down). To tell whether your estimate was correct (and your metabolism is functioning optimally), you should eat the required calories and monitor your weight weekly. Do this for one month. This will eliminate the weekly variances with water weight. If you gain weight, you're eating too much, so reduce your calories *slightly*. If you lose weight you're not eating enough, so increase your calories *slightly*. Keep doing this until a maintenance level is found. A word of caution: changes occur very slowly, so be patient.

RATIOS

After calorie level, the next most important factor to achieve your goals is the ratio between protein, carbohydrate and fat, and the response you get from your body.

The ratio between protein, carbohydrate and fat helps you regulate a powerful hormone: insulin. Insulin is a storage hormone. This means that when too much is present, calories will tend to be stored as fat. When something gets in to your system too quickly, such as a candy bar, there is a large amount of insulin released. Your body is set up to store calories then. Ideally, when you eat a meal, insulin levels will only be slightly elevated. Insulin also has an effect on hormones responsible for lean body mass gain.

The way your body handles proteins, carbohydrates and fats, and the type of response you get from insulin is primarily related to two genetic factors -- pH balance and the Autonomic Nervous System ANS.

Proteins and fats are very difficult to digest and require more of an acidic environment to be digested. Carbohydrates are easier to handle and are digested in a relatively alkaline environment. Everybody is born with their personal pH balance (neutral is 7.4). People who are more acidic (lower pH) tend to handle proteins and fats better. People who are more alkaline (higher pH) tend to handle carbohydrates better.

The other genetic factor, the Autonomic Nervous System, also plays a role. There are two parts to the ANS: the sympathetic and the parasympathetic. The sympathetic is the "fight or flight" response mechanism. A person who is sympathetic dominant has a lot of neural input going to the muscles, but less to the digestive organs. This person cannot handle the harder-to-digest items (proteins and fats), thus, carbohydrates are the preferred energy source.

The parasympathetic is the antagonist of the sympathetic. This person has a lot of neural input going to the digestive organs, rather than the muscles. The parasympathetic dominant person does better with a higher ratio of proteins and fats versus carbohydrates.

Everybody is born with a certain genetic make-up. For most people, a roughly 2:1 ratio of carbohydrate to protein and fat is needed to get the best response from the body (most fat loss and muscle gain). However, if a person is acidic and parasympathetic dominant, a higher percentage of protein and fat is required to get the best response (like a meat and potatoes person). Even at this extreme end, the amount of protein would be only *slightly* higher than the amount of carbohydrate and fat. At the other extreme is the alkaline person who is sympathetic dominant (your typical vegetarian). A good ratio for this person is roughly five times the amount of carbohydrate to protein and fat.

Getting too complicated? Don't worry. Start with the ratio that is best for most people: roughly 25 percent protein, 55 percent carbohydrate and 20 percent fat; your body will tell you the rest. If you eat an incorrect ratio for your system, you will release too much insulin and set your system up to store body fat. The feeling of wanting to curl up in a corner and fall asleep after a meal is a strong indicator of too much insulin, as is hunger or an unsatisfied feeling right after a meal. Sound familiar?

When you encounter either of these signs, the ratios need to be adjusted. Analyze the meal and see what the ratios look like. Depending on what you find, either add more carbohydrates, or proteins. See which gives you the most energy and a satisfied feeling. When eating in the correct ratio, cravings should be minimized because your body has what is needs. These ratios should be constant. Once you learn your ratios, if you desire weight loss or weight gain, you won't need to change your whole life. The only thing you will need to adjust are your calorie levels. Ratios will remain constant. You will stay leaner, recover quicker and have great energy all day - something we can all use.

SPACING

The last variable is the spacing of meals. To keep the metabolism high, you should eat at least every 2½ to 3½ hours. Eating small meals gives your system time to digest and assimilate the nutrients. If you continuously wait longer than 4 hours, your body thinks it is starving. At this point, your body starts to use your muscle for fuel, and releases enzymes responsible for storing body fat. So whether your goal is for weight gain or weight loss, the proper spacing of meals is critical.

In order to keep your overall calories in range, the total of all meals should equal the total calories required for the day.

To learn more about water, supplements, other key nutrients as well as sample menu plans, please get our book "The Final Edge-Peak Performance".

CHAPTER 4:
RESISTANCE EXERCISE

When considering an exercise program, remember: you can reach whatever goal you desire, no matter what equipment you use, as long as you are willing to put in the effort. In other words, it's not a certain machine or program that will get you there, it's your desire and effort. Of course, the right program or machine may enable to get there quicker.

The first step to putting it all together is remembering to warm up. Perform both a general and specific muscle-group warm up. The general warm up is intended just to get the blood flowing
all-over your body, and to raise your core temperature. This should take you about 5-10 minutes. The best warm up activities are those that use large muscle groups such as a stair-stepper or stationary bicycle; these machines don't require any bouncing movements which can overstretch and injure cold muscles. The specific warm up movements are performed after your core temperature is raised, but before a set of exercises. An example of a specific warm up is a light bench movement just before a set of chest exercises. Let's say your working weight is 25 pounds; your warm up weight might be 10 pounds.

Breathing is critical to proper lifting. You should never hold your breath longer than 1-2 seconds. On certain movements, a slight hold is needed to stabilize the motion (squats). As a rule, inhale when lowering, and exhale on the exertion. **The main point is to always breathe!**

FREQUENCY

Depending on your goals, the minimum commitment for resistance work is two days per week. The most you would need to commit is four days per week, with three days per week being optimal for most people. The only exception to this would be if you are peaking for a certain event or date. Then, for a limited time (2-3 months) before the event you would train up to 7 days per week. The factor to keep in mind is to do the best with what you have. So, if you can only make it 1 or 2 days in a week, don't worry. Shoot for 4 times the following week, or do extra on the weekend. *There is no magical formula*. Now, with realistic, achievable frequency goals in mind, remember that the other two variables of exercise are intensity and duration.

SPLITS
When you begin exercising, you will be able to get away with selecting just one exercise per muscle group, and working the entire body each workout session. However, as you progress, you will eventually want to add more exercises per muscle group and split the body up over two or more days depending on your goals and schedule.

The first step in setting up a routine is to decide how many days per week you can devote to an exercise program. You will need to divide your body so that each muscle group is worked directly or indirectly 2 times per week.

The next step is to define your priority areas. You should pick an extra exercise for this area and train it first in the routine when you have more energy, or train it alone on a separate day.

You can split the routines any way you want as long as no body part is trained on two consecutive days. One of the most popular ways to do this is the push-pull method. With this system you work all the pushing (chest, shoulders, quadriceps, triceps) on one day and all the pulling (hamstrings, back, biceps) on the next.

Other ways to split a routine would be chest and back on day one, legs on day two, and shoulders and arms on day three. You could work chest and triceps on day one, legs on day two, back and biceps on day three, and shoulders on day four. Keep in mind that when you work chest and back, you are also working your shoulders and arms quite a bit, so it's important to watch that the arms aren't getting trained with too many sets in one day.

Allow muscle groups time for recovery. Large muscle groups such as your back, chest and legs take longer to recover: 48-96 hours. Smaller muscle groups such as shoulders, arms, calves and abdominals require less time: 24-48 hours. Otherwise the types of splits are endless, anywhere from 2-7 days per week. Large muscle groups respond better to a heavy/light system, where one day per week they are hit hard, and the second time you hit them lighter with other angles.

<u>EXAMPLES</u>:

2 day split:

<u>Day 1</u>	<u>Day 2</u>
Inner/outer thigh	Front/back legs
Straight leg calves	Bent leg calves
Back	Compound shoulder & arms*
Chest	Abdominals
Abdominals	

3 day split:

<u>Day 1</u>	<u>Day 2</u>	<u>Day 3</u>
Back	Legs	Light back & chest
Chest	Calves	Arms
Inner thigh	Shoulders	Outer thigh
Abdominals	Abdominals	Abdominals

4 day split:

<u>Day 1</u>
Front/back legs
Straight leg calves
Shoulders
Abdominals

<u>Day 2</u>
Back
Chest
Abdominals

<u>Day 3</u>
Inner/outer thigh
Bent leg calves
Shoulders
Abdominals

<u>Day 4</u>
Light back/chest
Arms
Abdominals

*Compound shoulders and arm exercises include working the back and chest indirectly (i.e.: close-grip bench press) .

INTENSITY

After a complete warm up and warm up sets, every set should be taken to positive failure. This means you should keep performing repetitions until you cannot complete one more repetition in strict form. Every rep should be in continuous motion; do not stop and rest between reps as this lowers the intensity of the workout. The goal for intensity is to push to 100% for every set. Maximum effort will be different for you every time you work out. If you are low-energy on a given day, 100% may be half of the weight you typically use. Go with how you feel, and listen to your body.

REPETITIONS

Once you have the split decided, decide what repetition range you will use. A repetition (rep) is one complete movement (raising and lowering) of an exercise. The following continuum will be useful:

Rep continuum		
1-3 ___________________	12-15 ___________________	25+
strength	strength/endurance	endurance

To hit the various components of a muscle cell, your training must include reps all along the continuum at some point in your training. No matter what rep range you choose, when you get to the high end for reps, you will need to increase the resistance 2½ - 5 pounds (depending on the size of the muscle group). With this increase, you shouldn't be able to do all of the reps anymore. In order to progress, you must always ask your body to do more. When you increase weight, you are asking your body to do more.

A safe way to raise the intensity without raising the weight is controlling the speed of movement. Lift the weight so you can feel the muscle contract. Pause slightly, and lower it under control: roughly twice as slow as you raised it. This technique is safer than simply increasing the weight because the negative range of motion is stronger than the positive. Other ways to increase intensity without necessarily raising the weights are as follows:

<u>Forced reps:</u> having help to get past the sticking point and continue past failure. No more than 2-3 reps at the end of the set are ever needed.

<u>Cheating reps:</u> using momentum to get past the sticking point and continue past failure.

<u>Staggered sets:</u> performing an exercise in-between sets of the other exercises to increase volume for a muscle group.

<u>21's:</u> perform the bottom half of a movement for 7 reps, the top half of the movement for 7 reps, then the full movement for 7 reps.

<u>Descending sets:</u> after reaching failure, dropping the weight slightly to keep going. No more than three drops are needed.

<u>Negatives:</u> emphasizing the lowering of a movement.

<u>Manuals:</u> applying resistance to the movement to even out strength curves.

<u>Partial reps:</u> limiting the range of motion to be able to handle a heavier weight or continue past failure.

<u>Pyramiding:</u> starting with lighter warm up sets and increasing weight each set up to a peak, then working back down.

<u>Rest/Pause:</u> using a weight that allows for about 3 reps, resting for 5-15 seconds, performing 1-2 more reps, resting 5-15 seconds, performing 1-2 more reps, etc.

VOLUME

The more work you do the lower the intensity by definition. Performing endless reps and sets won't get you to your goals faster unless you raise the intensity. This is because muscles have a threshold.

With too much rest between sets, you won't break past the threshold and you won't progress. Practice resting 30-45 seconds between sets: just enough to catch your breath. The average number of sets (group of repetitions) you perform should be:

9-12 for large muscle groups (legs, back, chest)
6-8 for small muscle groups (shoulders, arms, calves, and abs)
You won't need more than 2-3 sets per exercise for a small muscle group and
3-4 sets per exercise for a large muscle group.

To learn more about recovery, overtraining, and get descriptions of how to perform key exercises, please get our book "The Final Edge-Peak Performance".

CHAPTER 5:
CARDIOVASCULAR EXERCISE

When considering a cardiovascular program, first determine what your main objective is, whether it's fat loss or cardiovascular conditioning. You can achieve both any time you perform aerobic activity, but the programs can differ with their *frequency* (number of times per week), *intensity* (effort), or *duration* (length of each session), depending on what your main goal is. Calorie expenditure can range from 200-500 calories for any given workout. This will be determined largely by the intensity and duration.

FREQUENCY

The minimum commitment for a cardiovascular program should be 3 times per week. Cardio can be performed up to 6 times per week because it is lower intensity than resistance work. It is always a good idea to take a day off per week for recovery. The more you can do (up to 6 days per week) the quicker your fat loss will be. Anything is better than nothing, so if you have severe time constraints, 1-2 days per week will lend you some results.

INTENSITY: TARGET HEART RANGE

The intensity is based on your maximum heart rate, or for a more accurate estimate, the Karvonen formula. Almost any activity will work for your goal. It is easier to work into your target heart range with large muscle groups working, such as stair climbing, walking or rowing.

Your target heart range (THR) is a percentage range of your maximum heart rate. THR has a minimum intensity threshold in order to be effective. THR also has an upper limit that when exceeded, leads into anaerobic activity. Two different methods to determine your optimal range are:

1. Maximum Heart Rate: Using the maximum heart rate method, take 220 minus your age and multiply by 65-90% to get you target heart range (the range, in beats per minute, your pulse should stay in during the activity).

2. Karvonen Formula: Using the Karvonen formula, take your maximum heart rate (220 minus your age) and subtract your resting heart rate (best if taken first thing in the morning, before getting out of bed). Multiply this number by 50-80% and add back in your resting heart rate.

FAT LOSS

Your optimal range for fat burning is much lower in intensity than you probably imagine. For fat loss use 50-60% for the Karvonen formula and 60-70% for the maximum heart rate formula for the intensity. This intensity is lower than the range for optimal cardiovascular benefits, but certainly best for fat burning. Duration is the most important factor. Always begin any program slowly, and build up the time gradually for safety.

CARDIOVASCULAR

For cardiovascular benefits use 60-80% for the Karvonen formula and 70-90% for the maximum heart rate formula for the intensity. Work at a lower intensity and a longer duration for fat loss because a greater percentage of the calories used are from fat. The longer the duration, the lower the intensity has to be, and the greater number of calories are burned from fat. Aerobic activity must be performed at least 20 minutes to be of benefit. As the intensity increases so does the percentage of calories used from carbohydrates. So, with a higher intensity you will burn more total calories in a given amount of time, but the calories burned will be primarily from glycogen (carbohydrate) rather than fat. If you're not as worried about fat loss, the higher intensity will get you into better cardiovascular condition.

DURATION

15 - 20 minutes is the least amount of time necessary to gain cardiovascular benefits. This is also the point where the body starts shifting the fuel source to fat as the primary source (instead of carbohydrates). The longer you continue past 20 minutes, the greater proportion of calories you burn will be from fat. The maximum benefit for fat burning is about 60 minutes, so we set this as the upper limit of the duration range. Remember that the total time with resistance and cardiovascular exercise should not exceed 1 ½ hours.

BEST OF BOTH

A good compromise between the two ends would be interval training. An intense, all out period is followed by a lower intensity period, followed by another intense period, followed by a lower intensity period, etc. The rest period is determined by your goals. A 1:3 work to rest ratio should be followed for people who need quick bursts of energy, while a 1:15 ratio would work better for longer endurance activities.

CHAPTER 6:
FLEXIBILITY

Flexibility is a key component of fitness, and should be performed every day. The chance of injury is much less if the joint is able to move through a full range of motion freely. Also, it enables you to develop maximum strength and size in a muscle, as you can work the muscle through a much greater range. I stress that you should **never stretch a cold muscle**. While stretching is a great warm-up, it should be preceded by at least five minutes of full body warm-up (bike, walking, etc.) to prevent muscle strains. You should also perform your stretches after exercise as a cool down.

TECHNIQUES

There are three main techniques to discuss: ballistic, static, and PNF (Proprio Neuromuscular Facilitation). **Ballistic** involves bouncing during the movement. This is the most dangerous type of stretching. There are receptors in every muscle that let it know when it is being stretched too far. When they sense that they are over-stretched, they signal the muscle to contract, as you know if you've ever fallen asleep in the car and your head snaps back. With ballistic stretching, it is easy to take the muscle too far. When this happens the muscle gets the signal to contract. As you can see, it is easy to strain the muscle if it is contracting while you are trying to stretch it.

Static stretching is the easiest and safest way to go. You simply hold each stretch for 30-60 seconds and repeat up to three times. Remember, however, not to over-stretch. Go just to the point of pain, back off slightly, and hold. If you try to go too far the muscle will actually end up tighter because of the receptors.

Proprio Neuromuscular Facilitation   (PNF) encompasses many techniques. I will discuss the most common. This technique will increase your flexibility the fastest, but a partner is usually needed. With this technique you are taken to a point of stretch by your partner. Hold this position for roughly a ten count, then hit an isometric contraction as your partner resists. This lasts for 8-10 seconds, and then your partner takes you to a greater stretch. This is done two to three times. By hitting the isometric contractions, you are fooling the receptors which allow for a greater stretch. This is also a great rehabilitative technique.

STRETCHES

While there are thousands of stretches and variations, here are my favorites for each major muscle group. Stretches should still be performed for the smaller muscle groups. Feel free to choose the stretches that you enjoy doing.

1. Quadriceps - Stand on the left leg. Use your left arm for balance. Bend the right leg up behind you and grab the right ankle with your right hand. Pull up and back until a gentle stretch is felt on the front of the leg. Repeat with the other leg. Use caution not to arch your back; keep your bent knee pointed downward toward the floor.

2. Hamstrings - Sit on the floor with your legs straight and feet together, keep a natural arch in the back, shoulder blades pinch back, and lean forward until a comfortable stretch is felt on the back of the legs.

3. Lower back - Lie with your back on the floor. Bring your knees to your chest. Pull on the legs from behind the knee (so you don't separate the knee). This can also be done with one leg extended.

4. Groin - Sitting on the floor with legs straight, separate the legs as wide as possible and lean forward while keeping the back in proper position until a comfortable stretch is felt on the inside of the legs. Keep toes pointed up toward the ceiling.

5. Hip - While sitting on the floor straighten both legs out in front of you. Bend the right leg up and cross it over the left leg. Twist the upper body to the right while pushing the right leg to the left until a slight stretch is felt in the right hip. Repeat with the other side.

6. Upper back - Find a post or something immovable to grab onto. Keep the knees slightly bent and pull back on the object. If stretching the right side, twist hips to the left and vice versa.
7. Chest/shoulder/bicep - Using a stick, grab out as wide as you can. Bring the stick over your head, directly behind the shoulders. For a greater stretch, bring the hands closer together.

8. Tricep - Bring the right arm up above your head and bend at the elbow so the hand is behind the head. With the left hand, apply pressure to the elbow and push the hand down the back until a slight stretch is felt. Repeat with the other side.

9. Calf - Facing a wall, stand back about 24 inches. Lean forward into the wall, keeping the legs straight and the heels in contact with the floor. This can also be done one leg at a time.